REVIEWS

"*Divine Birth* delivers an intimate, earthy and soulful collec▢ that holds reassuring messages, brings comfort, guides a▢▢▢▢▢▢▢▢▢ way! The freedom of expression and healing power of art beautifully complements the messages in the book!"
- Daphne Kostova, Author, Holistic Nutritionist, Model, Actress, mama of two

"I don't often feel myself smile upon opening a book, but the moment I started to explore Suzzie's work, my heart leaped for joy. She has woven a tapestry of past, present and future mother perspective, connecting spiritual wisdom with practical, empowering birthing advise. How I would have loved to have this book when I was pregnant and giving birth to my darlings. You can feel it energetically release fear and create an experience of love and alignment, within even the first few pages. Pure blissful delight!" A must read! - Love and light, Christina | www.spirituallyawareparenting.com

"In this inspiring book Suzzie Vehrs gently and lovingly nudges women away from the pain and fear often linked with childbirth and demonstrates that birth can take place in a space filled with support, love, empowerment, and breath. She not only carries women through the preparation for birth with her beautiful words and pictures but guides right through to the amazing moment of "I did it". The activity pages will be great preparatory exercises, birth-time empowerment tools and additions to a birth story memory book." - Christina Whelan-Chabot, Matters of Movement founder

"*Divine Birth* offers sage wisdom with a side of gentle encouragement. The beautiful illustrations and affirmations add to the calm, peaceful tone throughout the book. It's like reading a breath of fresh air!" - Sarah Cowan, Midwife Apprentice

"*Divine Birth* is a beautiful read with affirmations and images that empower women into a fearless birth." - Dorothy Guerra, Doula, Author of Yoga Birth Method

"Finding an outlet for the creative process going on within the human body is so important during pregnancy. This book is just that. You are adding powerful tools of self realization and belief into your toolbelt along the way. This is a place to put down your worries for a little while and come away knowing you are fully capable of doing what is to come." - Danie Crofoot, Full Spectrum Doula: Of Earth + Salt

"At a time when women all over the world are awakening to their power and taking back birth, they now have a beautiful guidebook to lead the way! Suzzie Vehrz's *Divine Birth* has the power to draw an expectant mother deep within herself and transform her into a confident and empowered birthing woman. Her beautiful images and thoughtful reflections draw the reader into a world of the Divine, bringing the mother to realize her value as a sacred life-giving vessel. Suzzie has a deep understanding that during the process of birthing a baby, a mother is also born. Delve deep into her meditative process, learn to trust in the way your body was created and experience the birth of your dreams!" - Maeve Ohrvall, Midwife, and Owner of Sacred Path Midwifery and The Birth Maven

"Giving birth is one of the most transformative experiences of a woman's life. Too often, our culture focuses solely on the physical process and neglects the necessary spiritual and emotional growth. This preparation is so important, regardless of what type of birth one is planning! Suzzie Vehrs's *Divine Birth* provides guidance and opportunity through a unique combination of activity and self-reflection. The drawings are rich with symbolism; encouraging contemplation while providing space for a woman to honor her emotions, focus her energies, release her fears and realize her full potential! The beauty and imagery of Suzzie's words are inspiring and empowering; and far beyond the typical birth affirmations." - Christine Sheets, Birth Worker, Educator and Reiki Master

"In *Divine Birth*, the beautiful Suzzie Vehrs brings together a powerful compilation of truths, stirring images, affirmations and relatable stories that illuminate the inherent power in every woman. A power that many of us don't realize we have, and cannot ever fully comprehend. But we can experience it. I devoured this book with a smile on my face the entire time because it captured SO MUCH wisdom about pregnancy and birth in such a concise and tidy package. I cannot wait to meditate on each of the beautiful illustrations as I color them with some fancy new pencils. This book is a gift for any woman who intends to birth a baby. I want all of the beautiful mamas in my community to read it! Thank you Suzzie for sharing your light with the world!" - Blair Fillingham, Founder/Chief Yogini, www.mtrnl.com | @blairfillingham

"Suzzie Stringham's *Divine Birth* is a collection of inspiration and grounding energy which will leave you totally empowered and prepared for the incredible journey that is motherhood. As the child is born, so is the mother, and the spiritual wisdom permeating these pages will help you reconnect with the immense power each of us women have as life-bringers." - Paulina Kapciak, Founder of New Generation Parenting and Mama Tribe

Divine Birth

A COLLECTION OF WISDOM + COLORING PAGES TO
INSPIRE AND EMPOWER THE PREGNANT MOTHER

DIVINE BIRTH: A COLLECTION OF WISDOM WITH COLORING PAGES TO INSPIRE AND EMPOWER THE PREGNANT WOMAN

2018 Golden Brick Road Publishing House Inc.
Trade Paperback Edition
Copyright @ 2018 Suzzie Vehrs

Published in Canada, Printed in China, for Global Distribution by
Golden Brick Road Publishing House Inc.
www.goldenbrickroad.pub

FOR MORE INFORMATION EMAIL: SUZZIEVEHRS@GMAIL.COM
ISBN: trade paperback 978-1-988736-47-1
ebook: 978-1-988736-48-8
Kindle: 978-1-988736-49-5
To order additional copies of this book: orders@gbrph.ca

Divine Birth

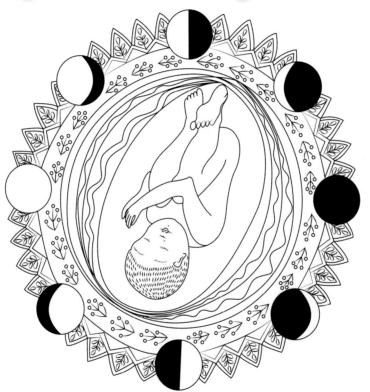

A COLLECTION OF WISDOM + COLORING PAGES TO
INSPIRE AND EMPOWER THE PREGNANT MOTHER

SUZZIE VEHRS

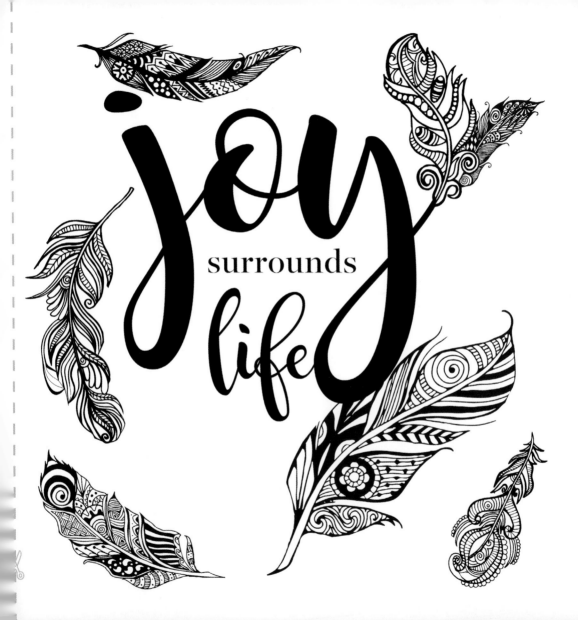

joy

surrounds

life

PREFACE

Birth has the potential to be the most transformative journey in a woman's life.

The moment a child is conceived in a woman's heart, the world is forever changed.

What if through birth, mothers around the world connected to their infinite value, immense power, and let go of every limitation and thought of self-doubt that has ever held them back?

Welcome to the *Divine Birth*. This book is designed to be a guide through which you give yourself a gift of reaching into your heart to uncover sacred truths about your capabilities and innate virtue as a woman, a mother, and a life bringer.

Full of birth wisdom, the words of this book will guide you as you begin your internal journey of looking within and finding yourself as a mother and creator of your birth. The pictures are there for you to fill with the depth, color, and emotion of your journey. As you spend time coloring, you give yourself time to be present with your emotions, feel into the space of your life changing, and prepare emotionally and spiritually for the journey of birth which you are about to embark on and transform through. When you have completed coloring the pages, you can hang them as a banner on the wall of your birthing area to remind you of the inner wisdom and power you have discovered within yourself through your birth preparations.

As you turn on your creative juices, you unleash that part of you that is no longer held captive by fear. You see that you can create beauty and bring a sense of magic and sacredness into your pregnancy and birthing experience.

During pregnancy, you are engaged in a sacred calling and process. Love yourself through it with infinite compassion as you unfold your own unique journey. Embrace the beauty of the moment, of the now. Allow this book to guide you as you move through your fear, embrace your deepest creative powers, and birth both yourself as a new woman and your baby into the world.

Each affirmation and symbol has a powerful meaning and the ability to activate different gifts and parts of your soul which will enrich your birth and allow you tap into the strongest, deepest parts of yourself. How would your birth be different if you **knew** you could do it? How would your life be different if you **knew** you were limitless?

"I am rooted but I flow."

- Virginia Woolf

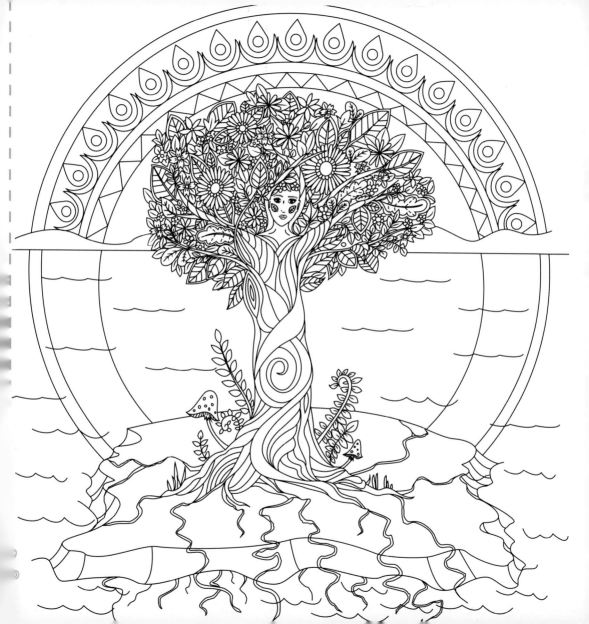

"I AM ROOTED BUT I FLOW." - VIRGINIA WOOLF

A beautiful thing about being human is this:
The opposites within endow us with great ability.

Our world is full of echoes of tales of birth being so painful that women need to be saved, and therefore there is only one right path, set before you by someone else. Or that birth is so sacred that all interventions should be avoided at any cost, despite what a woman wants for her own experience.

What if you could see these lies clearly for what they are, and the truth clearly for what it is?

It is impossible for a mother to fail. **Each and every type of birth is sacred. Especially yours. No matter how it unfolds.**

What if you **knew** that your world was safe?
Would that open the way for you to birth differently?
What if you **knew** that by sinking into your softness, your own power becomes available to be called upon as needed?

What if instead of allowing fear to keep you small in your dreams, you looked your fear in the eyes, turned on your intuition, and illuminated the perfect path for you? What would it take to move swiftly and freely forward down this path with both confidence and boldness?

If you seek strength, seek also softness.
If you seek clarity, understand the shadows of your deepest fears.
As you feel more power, prepare also to be aware of your vulnerability.
In all things, nurture the opposites within you.

For you already have everything you need to create the birth your soul is calling for.
You are so much more than a statistic.
You are unpredictable.

You are an outlier.
Out of nothing, you are creating a new body, a new soul, a new life.
Your powers to create are unlimited.
You have the power to treat your body as a temple of creation.
You have the power to find the most capable, attentive, and loving team for your birth.
You have the power to love yourself deeper and find more peace in your soul than you have ever had before.

In your soul lies the power to birth in *your* divine way.
In your soul lies the power to meet any challenges that present themselves to you along the way.

Repeat to yourself, "I am rooted, yet I flow."

Repeat to yourself, "I can do this."

Repeat to yourself, "I did it."

A woman's womb
is the most
sacred space
on the planet

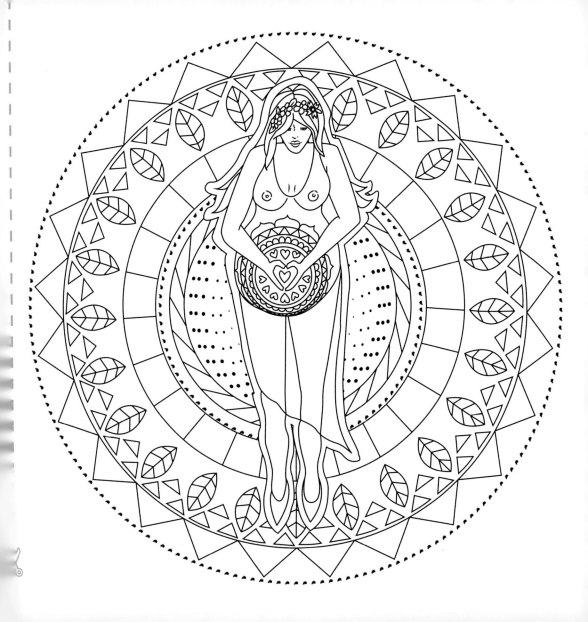

A WOMAN'S WOMB IS THE MOST SACRED SPACE ON THE PLANET

A woman's womb is the most sacred space on the planet. Within you, you have a child, growing, changing, becoming human. A spirit and a body are melding together, forming his or her impressions of the world. He or she is already eager to meet you, their carefully selected angel, earthside.

Know this: that **you do not ever have to give up your sense of feeling empowered in order to feel loved. Especially in birth.**

Your worth was determined before you were born, it is greater than the stars. Your beauty cannot be rated, diminished or lessened by what anyone else sees or does not see in you.

You were created by the Divine, and you have Divine within you. Therefore you are Divine. Because of this **you are limitless, powerful, beautiful, worthy, loved, cherished.**

You are released from all comparison, because all life has infinite virtue and value, especially yours. **Birth through the lens of infinite self-love.**

You are freed from shame as you know that no matter how your life has unfolded, you are on the perfect path for you. Your divinity is part of you and cannot be shaken. **Birth through the lens of infinite worthiness.**

You know that love is not earned. You cannot ever increase or decrease the amount of love available, for love is the very fabric by which the universe is tied together. All you have to do is open yourself to it. There is no reason to deny yourself that which you most deeply desire and no reason to stay small in hopes that you will be more loveable. The belief that you must choose between being loved and being yourself is one of society's greatest lies. **Birth through this lens, you are open to receive love and life in its purity and abundance.** The more love you allow into your life, the more love you allow into the lives of all those around you.

If you want more than what you have now in your birth vision, know that it is not guilt,

greed, or some unworthy part of you seeking these things, but your highest self bringing attention to the fact that more is available to you if you open yourself to it. **Birth through this lens, that all who surround you serve you as a human being, a sacred mother, and a divine creator.** You are not a medical problem gone wrong, you are a sacred and divine mother. Expect others to treat you as such.

Take time every day to honor your womb. It is your connection to the Divine Feminine, the Mother of all mothers, and our Mother Earth. *Who else could bring this specific life to the earth? No one. Only you.*

"How did you know you could do it?" they asked

"I looked within," she said

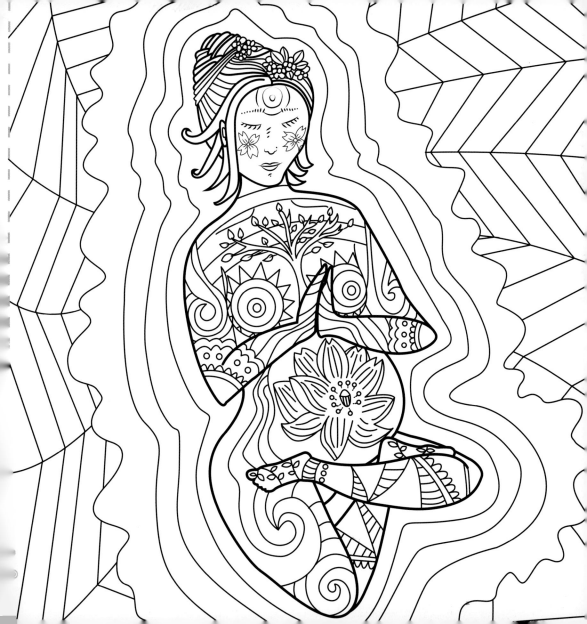

"HOW DID YOU KNOW YOU COULD DO IT?" THEY ASKED
"I LOOKED WITHIN," SHE SAID

When I was pregnant with my second child, I loved going to yoga. I chose to stay at my normal studio and modify as needed instead of going to a specific prenatal class during my first two trimesters. I loved the challenge and wisdom that was revealed to me within these classes. **Each class, like each birth, was a profound journey of self discovery.**

Often, when I would arrive to class, my mind would be full of excuses: *"Maybe I will skip most of class today because I am pregnant. Maybe I am too weak to do this. I am the only pregnant women here, I should take an easier path."* My mind would begin class full of reasons why I would "fail" before I even began.

As class picked up, and I began moving my body, I would feel my life force begin to move through me. My stagnation melted away. As the intensity picked up, **I would ask myself, "Can I do this?" And my body would respond, "Yes, can't you feel it?"**

The negativity that clouded my mind had to go away to make room for the new feelings that were filling me. Power, strength, awareness of the greatness that was the fabric of my soul. All of this flowed through me and became a part of me.

I loved feeling my breath sync with my body - one flow, one movement. I loved feeling my thoughts unite in strength. I particularly loved each moment where **I felt my weakness fall away from me. A shield that once protected me, no longer needed because it was my time to rise.**

My first birth reminds me of the beginning of a yoga class. My mind being full of untruths, yet believing them enough to allow them to guide me. I remember feeling, *"I don't think I*

27

can… I don't know if… I'm not meant for… I've failed…", as my birth unfolded in pain and self-depreciation.

I had yet to look in the mirror of truth and see what lies beneath the negative self-chatter. I hadn't yet found my core - the part of me that is limitless purely because it was fashioned by the Divine and not limited by my experience, my mother's experience, or a doctor's belief in me. I had missed the greatest journey of pregnancy, which is walking the path of discovery of one's truest, most sacred self.

By the time I entered labor the second time, I knew all I needed to birth this baby was already inside of me. All I had to do was look within.

Again I had the opportunity to face a task I was unsure of, and with each surge of pressure, sink deeper into my true being. I said goodbye to the part of myself that was filled with self-doubt over and over again, as each contraction passed, I saw that, **"I can do this because I am doing this."**

As each wave passed I sank into the knowledge of, **"I did it."**

Have you asked yourself, what lies inside of you? Pregnancy is the perfect nine months to embark on a path of self-discovery and find the magic that weaves your core.

What lies beyond your negative self-chatter? What makes you feel your life force pulsing through your veins and fills your body with certainty? **When you look in the mirror of sacred truth, what does it reveal about you that you don't take notice of and appreciate every day?**

When an "I can't…" or an "I'm not…" thought pops into your mind, remind yourself, "This is a lie that no longer serves me. I choose to think something else. I choose to see my true self now."

I can do this because I am doing this.

The strength, courage, and will to take your next step lies within you, even when all your internal reserves seem depleted and you feel unsure about your path.

Woven into your creation is wisdom, power, courage, love. These things will never leave you and will always guide you. Every accomplishment is made one step at a time. Do not worry about reaching the final destination, for it is certain that you will get there. During your birth, focus only on the contraction that is in front of you now, in this moment. You have every reason to know that in this moment, you can breathe through this contraction.

If you feel like you cannot do this anymore, move to a new space. Rotate between resting, eating, drinking, walking, dancing, being in the water, and being in your partner's arms. Allow your breath and movement to carry you through the early stages of labor until you truly, deeply, fully surrender to all that is and bring your baby earthside.

Birth is written in your DNA, your ancestors will whisper the path to you.

Someday, after this child is in your arms, someone will look at you and ask, *"How did you know you could do it?"* And you will respond, *"I looked within."*

i am
surrounded by
sacred support

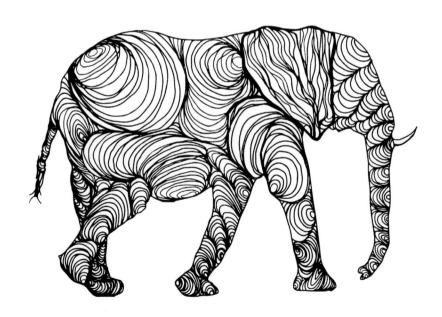

I AM SURROUNDED BY SACRED SUPPORT

Who is holding space for you to walk the unique path of your pregnancy and birth?

Elephants are a prime example of sacred sisterhood as they hold space for each other to safely bring life into the world. In the wild, when an elephant mother is in labor, if she is in any danger from nearby predators, fellow female elephants will surround the birthing mother and create a wall of safety around her as she brings her child earthside.

As you color this picture, ask yourself, **who is holding your sacred space as you are entering the most powerful and most vulnerable experience of you life?**

What does it mean to hold sacred space for someone? Holding space requires a person to put aside her own needs, ego, and desires in order to fully and completely serve you in whatever way you need. She must let go of her own predispositions of what you might need and give 100% of her presence, skills, and attention to walking alongside you without judgment. **She shares your journey to an unknown destination. She is completely and fully ready to go and do whatever you need from her.**

When someone holds space for you, it means they must completely dissolve their own ego, their own personal beliefs of what is right and wrong for you, and align with your inner wisdom. It means that they must see and hold sacred your deepest wisdom, and trust your journey and the lessons you will discover on your path.

Have you carefully selected a birth team that will walk with you this way?

What about your friends and family?

DIVINE BIRTH

A wonderful way to connect with your sacred sisterhood is to reach out to those who will not be at your birth, but who remind you of your divinity, value and capability. Send them each a candle and ask them to light it when you go into labor. While you are in labor, these sisters can pray, send you blessings, and hold you in safety and security.

All you need to do is look at this picture to be reminded that **you are surrounded by a sacred sisterhood,** composed of both those on earth whom you love and angels surrounding and attending to you. However your path unfolds, you will be fully supported and completely protected as you enter this path of self-discovery and birth.

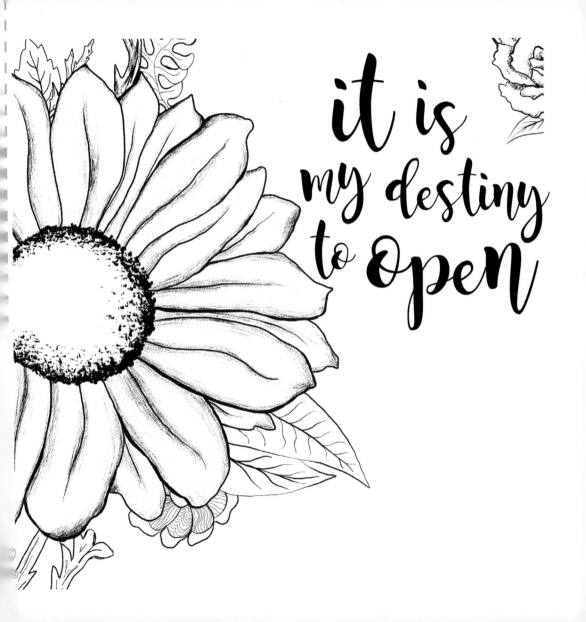

IT IS MY DESTINY TO OPEN

Just as a flower blooms open and wide, *it is your destiny to open to allow life to flow through you* to join us earthside. Now is the time to let go of all the stories of pain, fear, and doubt that tend to surround pregnancy and birth. Humans are the only species that doubt their ability to birth. It is tension and tightness that arises from doubt and fear which turns the intensity of labor into pain during the birthing process. Allow yourself to melt into labor, understand that intensity is a gift. It will all end, your baby will be in your arms. **Your body is designed to birth, and it will open.**

Remember, **a pressure wave cannot be stronger than you for it *is* you.** Each wave is your body and your baby moving with purpose towards life. Allow, surrender, enjoy.

As you color this image, ponder the ways you can open and soften to life in your world today. Are there places where you are holding onto pain because that is what everyone else is doing? Send those feelings deep into the core of Mother Earth and allow her to transmute them into the confidence of knowing with surety that you have been perfectly designed to birth in joy.

As every pressure wave washes through you, sink into the knowledge that you are opening deeper and deeper physically, emotionally, and spiritually to the Divine love which supports you at every moment.

Now is your time to open to life. Sink into trust and embrace all that makes your life feel magical. Life is flowing through you and out of you. **It is already written in the stars. It is your destiny to open.**

SUZZIE VEHRS

The gift
of Intensity
is Immense
Intimacy

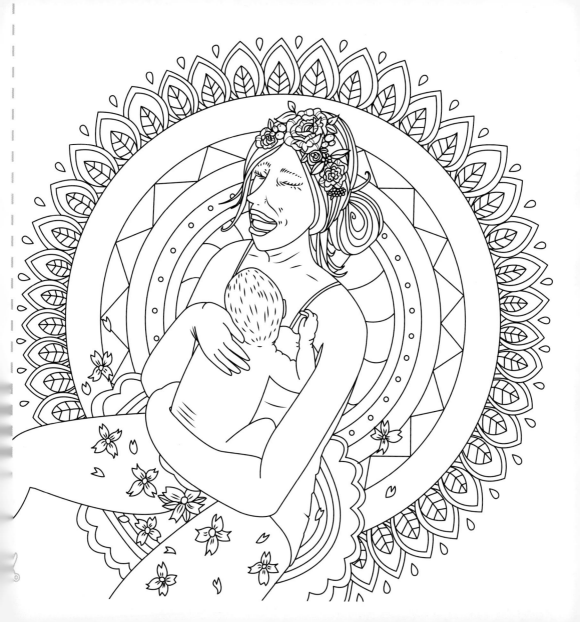

SUZZIE VEHRS

THE GIFT OF INTENSITY IS IMMENSE INTIMACY

How will that first moment feel when your baby is in your arms, at your breast, staring up at you with their big wide eyes for the very first time?

This very moment is the one destined for you. You have no reason to doubt that it is possible and no reason to doubt your ability to get here.

Yes, **you will be challenged in the process of bringing your baby earthside. Like a woman emerging from the most significant quest of her life, like a butterfly emerging from its chrysalis, you are destined for greatness.** May all that is not aligned with your highest self, or your greatest possibilities for this birth, be shaken from you through this journey.

The gift of intensity is that it brings an immense intimacy. Forever. That is how long you are tied with this child. Forever in each others hearts. Forever is how long your souls are tied together in love and service to one another.

Know that you are enough. You are everything this child needs.

One of my favorite Law of Attraction teachers, Abraham Hicks, speaks of how if you can hold something in your mind for seventeen seconds, you plant a seed that can and will emerge. Spend time every day, even if it is only a few seconds, to envision this first moment with your child. Hold the surety, the joy, the elation, the immense intimacy, the flood of rightness of being together, in your mind.

Sink into the feeling of knowing how good it will feel to to hold your child in your arms for the first time, baby's skin perfectly soft against yours. How amazing will the first newborn

43

smell be? How precious those tiny little fingers and toes. What about that first tug at your breast? And that feeling of being infinitely aware of the heavens opening to allow this child their experience on earth.

Allow your heart and your mind to reside in this moment, even before it happens. Whisper the stories of this moment to your growing baby often before he or she is here. Call these images like warriors to the front of your memory as your labor intensifies. This vision will sustain you as you and your child work together through labor.
Mother, you've got this! **Your baby will be here soon.**

Focus on the exhale and the inhale will take care of itself

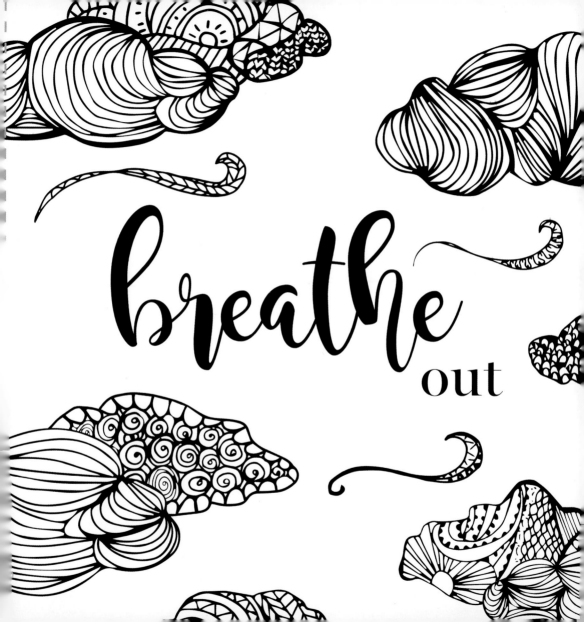

breathe

out

FOCUS ON THE EXHALE AND THE INHALE WILL TAKE CARE OF ITSELF

In Ayurveda, ancient Indian medicine, there are five elements: Earth, Water, Fire, Air, and Ether (self). Earth gives us stability, Water allows serenity and flowing, Fire creates change, and Air, the lightest element, brings movement.

Unseen yet ever present, the Air element prepares us to accept the fifth and final element, Ether, self, or spirit. It helps us believe that something doesn't have to be seen to be real and gives us the faith needed to feel into our spirit and soul where true, innate wisdom lies. It is here that your personal blueprint to birth is discovered, not anywhere else.

It is from this space, between the movement of all your thoughts, that **you _know_ you can birth because in your heart it has already been done.**

Every breath, every pressure wave, brings more certainty that your baby will be in your arms soon.

Have you ever noticed when you become stressed or tense you hold your breath as if time would stop if you just held it in? If you haven't noticed this yet, pay attention. Remember this: **tension cannot exist where air is flowing.**

If breathing ever seems forgettable, **_focus on the exhale and the inhale will take care of itself._** The more oxygen you gently breathe out of your system, the more life-giving air will fill your lungs automatically. Your body is magical that way.

Slow down, focus on the exhale, and breathe your baby out.

To practice this before your baby is here, find a simple feather and blow it lightly across the room. If you already have kids, they will *love* joining you in this as you dance to your favorite music. This is the kind of breathing that will allow you to loosen, release, and allow your baby to move through you.

To help your birthing body open, you can also repeat the words, *"Open,"* or *"Yes."* Another simple focus point is repeating the ancient Sanskrit word *"Om."* Translated to modern day English, Om is understood as the breath of life, or life's first breath. Repeating this sound will bring you the lightness you need to move and birth with ease.

An ancient Indian teacher, Pantajali, is quoted as saying, "Chant Om and you will attain your goal. If nothing else works, just chant Om." Whether you chant, roar, or moan, let out this sacred word whenever you need it and feel your baby move towards her first breath of life in your arms.

I am one with
the source
of creation and
all mothers
everywhere

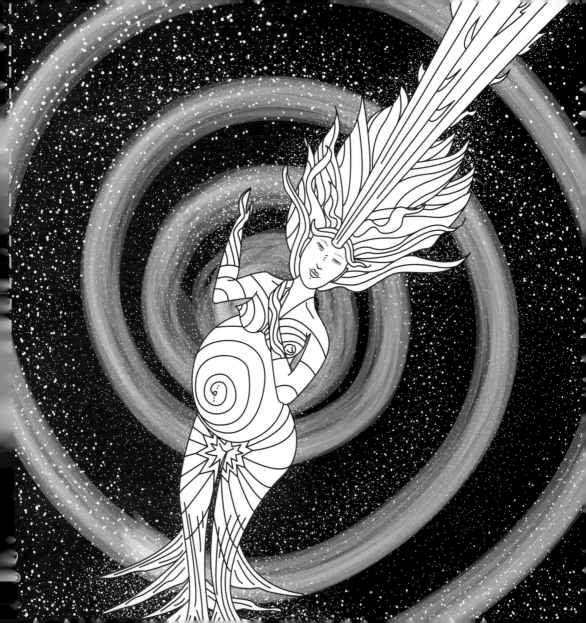

I AM ONE WITH THE SOURCE OF CREATION AND ALL MOTHERS EVERYWHERE

Light in the darkness. Peace in the confusion. Roots when everything is shifting. At one time or another, you may feel like you cannot do this anymore. Yet there is a candle burning in your soul, so powerful it can eradicate any darkness.

You will see clearly. You will feel peace. Your heart and mind will unify. **You will know the way because it is already inside of you.**

When you get to the point where you feel defeated and cannot go on, this is the moment when you have the ability to become one with the the source of creation, the Divine Mother, and all mothers birthing with you at this time.

Summon the power of this collective to you. **Let divine ability vibrate through every molecule of your being and every cell of your body.** Every wave of power has brought you deeper and deeper within yourself, to a place where you can fully surrender and become one with all mothers.

Within the place of uncertainty is where you decide that you will commit and move forward. This is where you leave behind the old you and emerge as the new you, the mother of this child. You are fully capable, no longer doubting if you can handle the tasks before you.

You are a powerful creator. You have everything within you to bring life to this world. **Miracles are your birthright. Angels surround you in this moment.**

Your roots are deep, pulling in love and capability.**You are fully aware of the divine strength coursing through your body, the full power of creation transforming you**

into everything you thought you could not be, as it moves your baby through your body.

You are now **MOTHER,** creator and sustainer of life. You are part of the divine force of creation. She is you and you are her, totally inseparable.

At this moment when your body and soul have opened more than it has ever done before, you know all things. Now allow your roots to nourish you and receive.

Receive peace, sanctuary, safety at the top of the mountain. The triumph of love over all. Allow yourself to be meditative, not strained, for you are gaining the interior knowledge that you can, you will, and you did bring this child to earth. **This is the place where the strength of the universe and every mother who has ever done this before will fill your soul, wash through you, and endow you with a power that you never had before.**

You can stop struggling, because now through this great power that is not yours, but is you and every mother who has ever been, you will do one thing. You will surrender and allow the Divine Mother to take you the rest of the way. Just as you will cradle your baby in your arms, she cradles you now. You have the courage, the power, to stand by your core and truest self in this birthing moment. Remember what matters and forget everything that does not.

This baby is coming to you now.

I am free to birth my way

I AM FREE TO BIRTH MY WAY

As you complete this book, you have spent time examining your fears, you have quieted the monologues of doubt and shame that fill the atmosphere which we breathe, and found value in your own unique journey and birthing experience. You are connected to that part of you which is not ego, that part of you which is connected to all of life, that part of you which is connected to divine wisdom and direction. **You have practiced being present and you have mastered calling the joy and sacred wisdom into your being. You have learned to trust your innermost voice. You are now free birth in your own way.**

As a sacred mother, in the act of creating and birthing a baby, you are eternally safe and protected as your most authentic self. In this place of freedom, **you are endowed with limitless raw power.** Your safety comes from your strength which has always been within you, which you can now feel pulse through your veins.

Let the lion remind you that your highest self is calling you to your life's greatest possibility for this birth. **Let your vision roar through you, your family, your space, and all who enter your space.** Your sacred vibration will shake away any and all selfish and impure motives of those around you.

As you embrace your inner power and the power of the Divine that flows through you, you are released from tension and allowed to **sing with joy, dance under the light of the moon, embrace your playfulness, and move your hips as you labor down this child.** At any moment, your fierceness is ready to be called upon and exercised, which is exactly the knowledge you need to release, relax, and dance into the flow of birth.

Have you ever wondered if birth can be positive, or even enjoyable?
The answer is yes. Just ask these mothers:

"I'm addicted to giving birth!! I love every bit of power and strength. It's raw, powerful, and life changing! It's all about your mindset and how you perceive birth. A positive mind is a sure winner for a positive birth." - Mandy Lynn

"I look back on it with soooo much happiness and pleasure . I do remember there was a lot of pain (I had intense back labor), but my overall feeling throughout it all was peace, serenity, love. My mindset going in was that pain is temporary and I can deal with any level of pain because it is temporary. I also never truly believed or felt like I was in labor - the idea of labor was so big in my head, I never felt like I reached it. The entire time, I was thinking, "This is great, this is manageable, more/worse pain is coming..." and then the worse pain never came because I was through transition. I'm not sure that even makes sense, but it was just an awesome, surreal experience for me that I look back on fondly." - Heidi Martinez

"I have a couple of babies that I literally laughed out." - Jennifer Bowman

Hear this: In an analysis of factors thought to influence labor pain which include fear of pain, confidence, concern about the outcome of labor, frequency of contractions, menstrual pain, and size of baby: **confidence consistently emerged as the most significant predictor of pain for the entire time a woman's cervix is dilating.** Confidence in yourself means less pain and a simpler birth.[1]

The path to the best birth does not lay outside of yourself, but within yourself. If you are ready to birth yourself and your child, together, as powerful whole beings, you must look within.

Remember these four ways that you as a mother can cope with and move the power of creation through your body as you and your baby work together to bring this new life earthside.

1. *Relax into yourself between pressure waves.*
2. *Vocalize your needs and release pain with moans, the word "yes," or the word "open."*
3. *Exhale breath and tension.*
4. *Hold tightly to your vision of the moment at the end of the journey where your baby will be in your arms. Communicate positive words of this moment to your child as you progress.*

How you feel about your capabilities is one of the most important factors determining your experiences in birth and life. Know you are powerful enough to do this. **Dare to look into the mirror of truth, and discover that at the core of your being, you are infinitely capable.** You are enough in every way. Your birth, in all it's uniqueness and beauty, is enough in every way, exactly how it is written in your experience.

Birth through your authenticity and your life with change.

You are not meant to live someone else's story, but to unfold your own divine and unique journey.

You are a more capable creator than you dare to imagine.

Trust yourself and know that however your story unfolds, it will guide you to your highest light.

You can do this!

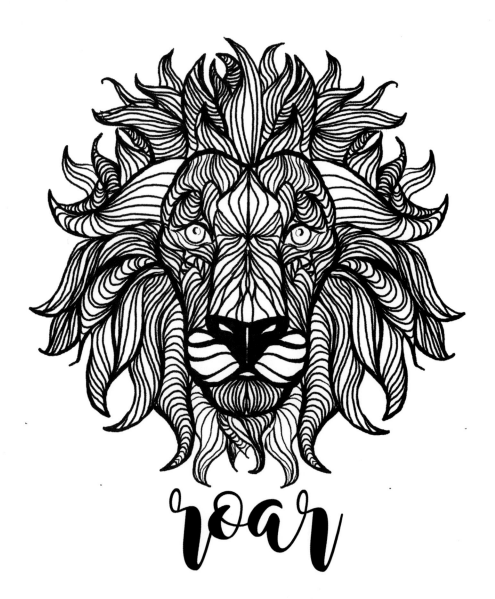

I did it

CREATE YOUR OWN

On the following pages, you will find beautiful mandalas, frames and blank pages. As you color these, add in any sayings or quotes that will help you surrender to your own birth. You may also add images of your family, ultrasound pictures, or anything else that will help you focus and open as you birth your baby.

Would you like some inspiration?

I asked a group of new mothers which affirmations were the most powerful for them during birth, and this is what they said. Feel free to use these or create your own. The space here is yours to create.

"Women around the world are doing it with me."

"Surrender to the process."

"Let your monkey do it." - Ina May Gaskin

"Let it be."

"One at a time."

"Ride the wave."

"She will be here soon."

"This too shall pass."

"The moment I'm ready to quit is the moment right before baby is here."

"I can handle anything for 10 seconds. 1, 2, 3, 4, 5, 6, 7, 8, 9,10." Repeat.

"This is it, there is no alternative. Mind over matter. I'm doing this."

"Just keep moving forward. This is all working for my baby. I know the reward."

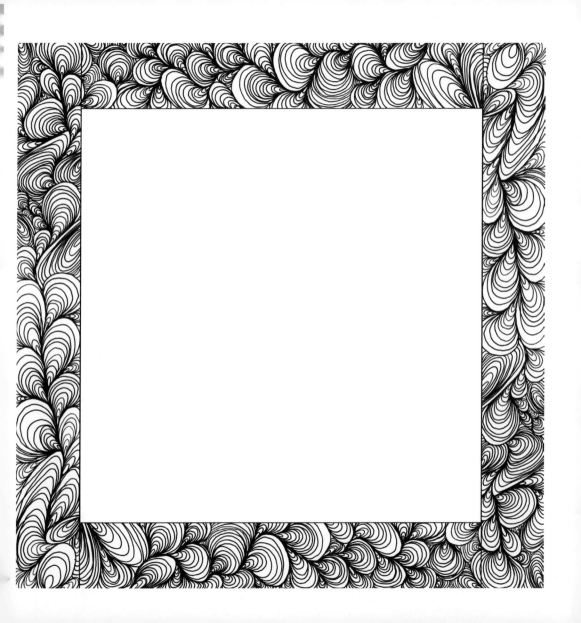

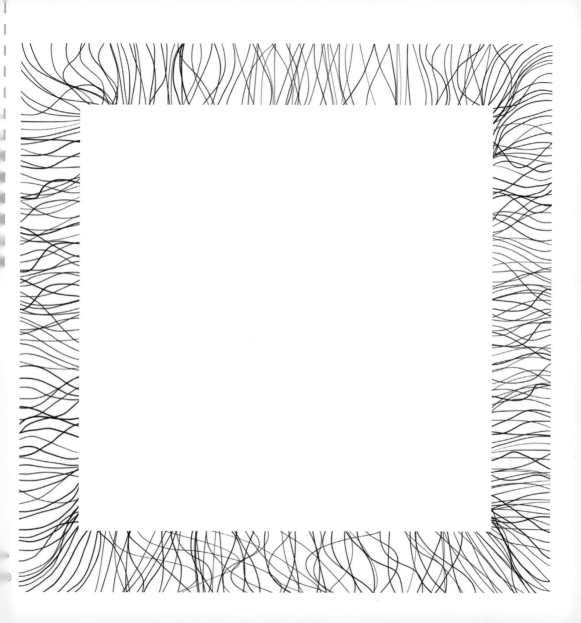

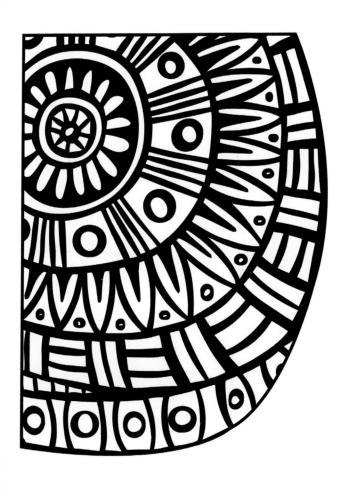

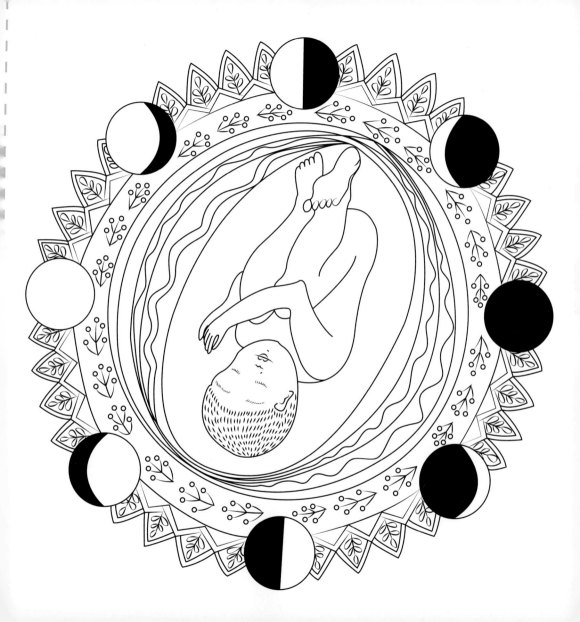

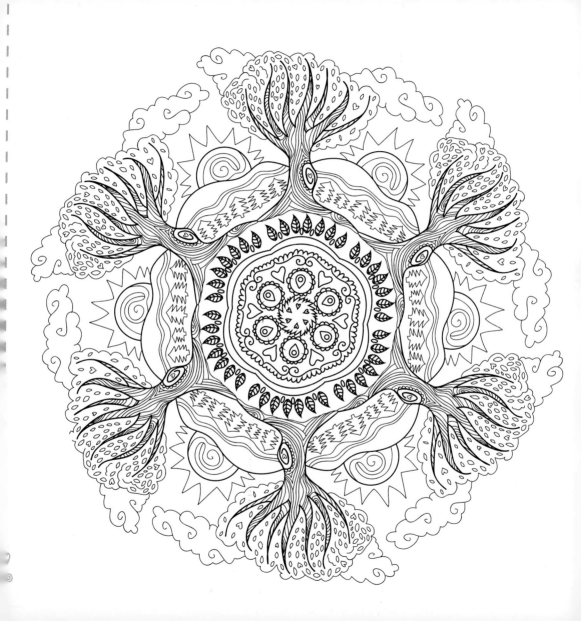

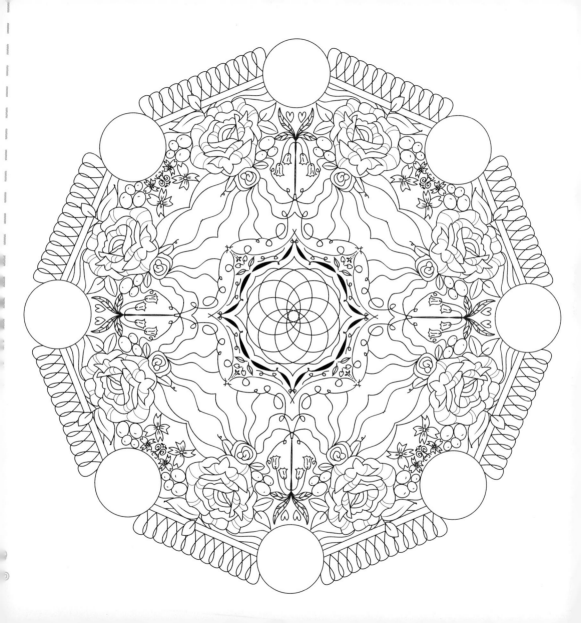

REFERENCES:

Bachman, Margo Shapiro. Yoga Mama, Yoga Baby: Ayurveda and Yoga for a Healthy Pregnancy and Birth. Sounds True, Inc., 2013.

Bartlett, Whapio D. "Holistic Stages of Birth." The Matrona, www.thematrona.com/the-holistic-stages-of-birth/

Gaskin, Ina May. Birth Matters: a Midwife's Manifesta. Seven Stories Press, 2011.

Lowe, N. (2002, May). The name of labor pain. American Journal of Obstetrics and Gynecology, 186, 256.

Miller, Daniel. "Try Getting Past This Lot! Elephants Huddle Round Female to Protect Her from Prowling Hyenas While She Gives Birth." Daily Mail Online, Associated Newspapers, 29 Feb. 2012, www.dailymail.co.uk/news/article-2108183/Herd-elephants-huddles-round-female-gives-birth.html.

Tornetta, Giuditta. Painless Childbirth: an Empowering Journey through Pregnancy and Birth. Cumberland House, 2008.

Webster, Bethany. "Why It's Crucial for Women to Heal the Mother Wound." Womb of Light, www.womboflight.com/why-its-crucial-for-women-to-heal-the-mother-wound

SUZZIE VEHRS,
AUTHOR

Suzzie Vehrs is a mother, writer, economist, and birth educator. The loss of her first pregnancy and the traumatic experience with the birth of her first child left her shattered. However, her path to healing and reclaiming her life led her to uncover and rediscover beautiful truths about motherhood, life, and birth that had long been hidden to her and have made the journey all worthwhile. She teaches mothers how to embark on a powerful journey of self-discovery through pregnancy and birth in authentic ways that serve each person's unique needs. Every woman is capable of birthing not just a baby with a measurable pulse, but a life that pulses with vibrance and beauty at the same time.

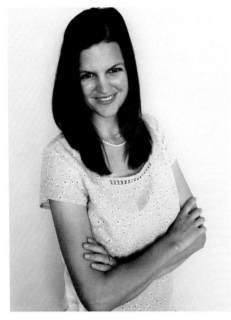

To connect with Suzzie, download free pregnancy affirmations or find out more about her birth preparation class visit: www.moregigglingmoments.com

or follow her on instagram @moregigglingmoments

REGAN HOWARD,
ILLUSTRATOR

Regan is a spiritual empath, epressive healer, and intuitive light-worker. She is a life-long creative that is full of compassion and support. She is the creator of Hue & You, a high-vibe company rooted in allowing women to work through their experiences in an expressive fashion where no words are ever needed. The striking style and passionate nature of her company and programs allo her students to embrace their journey, receive self-empowering techniques, and give them the guidance to live their truth fearlessly!

JESSICA DEAKEN,
ILLUSTRATOR & GRAPHIC DESIGNER

Jessica Deaken is a Multidisciplinary Artist - Fine Art, Illustrations, and Graphic Design. Born in open, artsy Montreal, Quebec, spending half of her earlier years there and moving out West to beautiful British Columbia with her family at age eleven. Jessica grew up in BC embracing natures beauty, around her always. She moved back to study Art and Design for four years in her late twenties; re-discovering her roots in beautiful, European, friendly, charming, Montreal. Jessica always finds herself taking moments to embrace the simple Zen moments, like the smell of flowers, the picturesque landscapes, or the sequence of how plants grows, and the laughter of her children, because in all the madness there are beautiful moments. After studying she moved back to BC, and as of July 2018 has been residing in Ontario. You can find her creating large scale Contemporary Abstract paintings, creating illustrations for books, book layout design, or into some other aspect of Art & Design. Jessica loves bringing her clients dreams to life, often trying to find ways to pack meaning into her art pieces, however leaving some mystery, so, up for interpretation. She feels that evoking an emotion from the art she creates is very important, and will often fall in love with her own art pieces.

Jessica is often open to new artistic endeavours,
contact Jessica through email: jessica.deaken@gmail.com

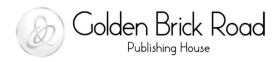

Golden Brick Road
Publishing House

Locking arms and helping each other down
their Golden Brick Road

At Golden Brick Road Publishing House, we lock arms with ambitious people and create success through a collaborative, supportive, and accountable environment. We are a boutique shop that caters to all stages of business around a book. We encourage women empowerment, and gender and cultural equality by publishing single author works from around the world, and creating in-house collaborative author projects for emerging and seasoned authors to join.

Our authors have a safe space to grow and diversify themselves within the genres of poetry, health, sociology, women's studies, business, and personal development. We help those who are natural born leaders, step out and shine! Even if they do not yet fully see it for themselves. We believe in empowering each individual who will then go and inspire an entire community. Our Director, Ky-Lee Hanson, calls this: The Inspiration Trickle Effect.

If you want to be a public figure that is focused on helping people and providing value, but you do not want to embark on the journey alone, then we are the community for you.

To inquire about our collaborative writing opportunities or to bring your own idea into vision, reach out to us at:

www.goldenbrickroad.pub

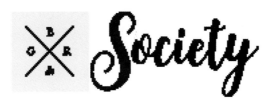

Goals, Brilliance, and Reinvention

Join us at the social

www.gbrsociety.com

GBR Society is a community of authors, future authors, readers, and supporters. We are connected through Golden Brick Road Publishing House; a leadership, empowerment, and self-awareness publisher. The GBR empire is built on sharing opportunity. It is a brand built on being a true community consisting of friendship, allies, support, advancing with each other, philanthropy, and tribe work. We struggle together and we flourish together. We are a community budding with endless ongoing love. Get to know the real people behind successful author brands and careers. Build friendships with motivated people and find your own voice. We have been said to be guides in helping others discover their own strength.

Join us as a reader and gain a wealth of insight from our authors and featured guests, while receiving access to exclusive advanced books, online and in person events, bookclubs, summits, online programs, retreats, and special offers. Learn from us how to advance in your personal and professional life. Access information on what interests you, choosing from health and wellness, sociology, human rights, writing and reading, creating a business, advancing a business or career, and personal development including self-esteem, introspection, self-discovery, and self-awareness.